Ketogen Cookbook

Recipes Low in Carbohydrates
to Encourage Healthy Living
with Easy-to-Follow, Quick,
Delicious, and Keto-Friendly
Meals

By

Emily William

strictly prohibited and any storage of this document is not allowed unless with written permission from the publisher. All rights reserved.

The information provided herein is stated to be truthful and consistent, in that any liability, in terms of inattention or otherwise, by any usage or abuse of any policies, processes, or directions contained within is the solitary and utter responsibility of the recipient reader. Under no circumstances will any legal responsibility or blame be held against the publisher for any reparation, damages, or monetary loss due to the information herein, either directly or indirectly.

Respective authors own all copyrights not held by the publisher.

The information herein is offered for informational purposes solely, and is universal as so. The presentation of the information is without contract or any type of guarantee assurance.

The trademarks that are used are without any consent, and the publication of the trademark is without permission or backing by the trademark owner. All trademarks and brands within this book are for clarifying purposes only and are owned by the owners themselves, not affiliated with this document.

Table of Contents

Introduction

The ketogenic diet is a diet in which carbohydrates are reduced to less than 50 grams per day, with a relative increase in proteins and fats.

For many years, the low-carbohydrate diet has been used to cure epileptics. It is even mentioned in the Bible (New Testament, Matthew 17: 14-21).

Ketosis is a rather misunderstood metabolic state that generates many fears.

Is the Ketogenic Diet the Same as the Paleolithic or Atkins Diet?

The original Atkins diet was developed in 1960 and is considered a ketogenic diet. Currently, the Atkins diet has undergone modifications and is called Atkins New Low-Carb Experts, where they offer an initial plan of 20 grams of carbohydrates per day, using processed products such as sunflower oil, Atkins bars, canola oil, among others. Then, in the following phases, the suggested carbohydrate values are raised.

The Paleolithic diet is more of a dietary model than a single diet. This model is based on the inclusion of natural foods, those consumed by man in the Paleolithic era, a period ranging from 3 million to 12 thousand years BC. The hunter-gatherer diet includes foods such as wild animals, grazing animals, wild animals, fruits and vegetables, seeds, nuts, mother's milk. It does not include processed, diet or light products, oils, dairy products and the only beverage included is water. This food model in itself suggests not to abuse fruits (which would be the sources of sugars in the diet) because the primitive man only found fruits from time to time.

Herein lies the difference since neither fruits nor vegetables are restricted as in a ketogenic diet where the premise is the reduction of sugar sources, including fruits.

Does a Ketogenic Diet Reduce More Kilos Than a Traditional Diet?

Several studies have shown that the ketogenic diet is more effective for weight loss than low-calorie diets.

The mechanisms by which the ketogenic diet is more effective for weight loss are:

1. By reducing dietary carbohydrates, blood insulin decreases, this deactivates lipogenesis (which means accumulating fat).
2. For 1 to 3 days, the sugar reserves found in the liver and muscles are used.
3. The Nervous System picks up this situation and sends signals to obtain

glucose through the burning of fats from the adipose tissue in the liver (lipolysis).

4. The fats in the liver are converted into ketone bodies which are substances capable of offering their energy to the tissues, especially to the brain.

5. Fats are also converted into glucose to maintain acceptable blood glucose levels.

6. Many of the ketone bodies are eliminated by evaporation through respiration, which leads to loss of energy (fat lost through the breath). They are also eliminated in the urine.

Chapter 1. Smoothies & Breakfast Recipes

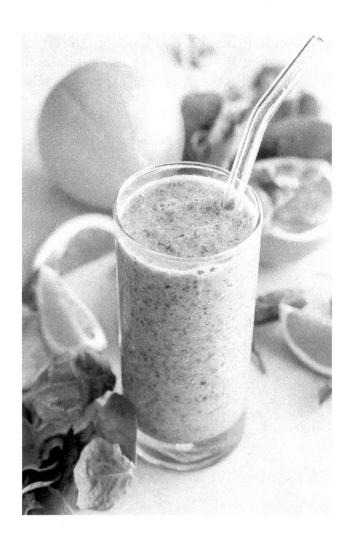

Smoothies
1. Keto Green Smoothie

Ready in about 5 min | serving 1 | Difficulty: Easy

Per serving: Kcal 341, Fat: 24.7g, Net Carbs: 25.1g, Protein: 5.6g

Ingredients

- Spinach blend 2/3 cup (20g)

- Avocado 1/2 medium

- MCT oil powder 1 scoop (10g)

- Pure vanilla extract 1 tsp

- Matcha powder 1/2 tsp

- Golden monk fruit sweetener 1 tbsp (12g)

- Coconut milk 1/2 cup (120ml)

- Water 2/3 cup

- Ice cubes

Instructions

1. Mix all ingredients and blend until well-combined.

2. Chocolate Fat Bomb Smoothie

Ready in about 5 min | serving 1 | Difficulty: Easy

Per serving: Kcal 276, Fat: 26.2g, Net Carbs: 31.2g, Protein: 2.7g

Ingredients

- Ice cubes 2

- Unsweetened coconut milk ½ cup (120ml)

- Coconut cream ¼ cup (60g)

- Fruit sweetener 2 tbsp (24g)

- MCT oil powder 1 scoop (10g)

- No-sugar-added Sun butter 1 tbsp (16g)

- Unsweetened cocoa powder 1 tbsp (5g)

- Salt 1/16 tsp

Instructions

1. Mix all ingredients and blend until well-combined.

3. Golden Smoothie Keto

Ready in about 5 min | serving 1 | Difficulty: Easy

Per serving: Kcal 210, Fat: 19.1g, Net Carbs: 18.3g, Protein: 0.4g

Ingredients

- Canned coconut cream ¼ cup (60g)

- MCT oil powder 1 scoop (

- Freshly grated ginger 1 tbsp (~7g)

- Golden monk fruit sweetener 1 tbsp (12g)

- Ground turmeric ¾ tsp

- Pure vanilla extract ½ tsp

- Black pepper ⅛ tsp

- Cinnamon ⅛ tsp

- Ice cubes 4

- Cup water ¼ cup + 2 tbsp divided

Instructions

1. Mix all ingredients and blend until well-combined.

Breakfast
4. Keto Scrambled Eggs with Halloumi Cheese

(Ready in about 20 mins |Serving 2| Difficulty: Easy)

Per serving: Kcal 657, Fat:59g, Net Carbs:4g Protein:28g

Ingredients

- Olive oil 2 tbsp

- Diced halloumi cheese 3 oz

- Chopped scallions 2

- Diced bacon 4 oz

- Chopped fresh parsley 4 tbsp

- Eggs 4

- Salt & pepper

- Pitted olives 2 oz

Instructions

1. Heat olive oil in a frying pan over med-high, and cook scallions, halloumi, and bacon until well browned.

2. Whisk the parsley, the eggs, salt & pepper together in a tiny cup.

3. The egg mixture is poured over the bacon & cheese into the frying saucepan. Reduce the gas, add the olives and then mix for a few minutes.

5. Keto Pancakes with Berries and Whipped Cream

(Ready in about 25 mins |Serving 4| Difficulty: Easy)

Per serving: Kcal424, Fat:39g, Net Carbs:4g Protein:13g

Ingredients

Pancakes

- Eggs 4

- Cottage cheese 7 oz

- Husk powder ground psyllium 1 tbsp

- Butter 2 oz

Toppings

- Fresh raspberries 2 oz

- Heavy whipping cream 1 cup

Instructions

1. In a medium-size dish, incorporate the eggs, psyllium husk, and cottage cheese and blend. Let sit for 5 to 10 mins to thicken.

2. Heat a non-stick skillet with butter or oil. Fry on either side of the pancakes at med-low heat for 3

to 4 minutes. Don't make them so wide, or they'll be tough to turn over.

3. Add the cream and whip to a separate bowl until the soft peaks form.

4. Serve.

6. Keto Deviled Eggs

(Ready in about 15 mins |Serving 4| Difficulty: Easy)

Per serving: Kcal 163, Fat:15g, Net Carbs:0.5g Protein:7g

Ingredients

- Eggs

- Tabasco 1 tsp

- Mayonnaise ¼ cup

- Herbal salt 1 pinch

- Cooked & peeled shrimp 8

- Fresh dill

Instructions

1. Begin by boiling the eggs in a pot and then with water covering them. Position the pot and bring to a gentle boil over med heat.

2. Boil for 8 to 10 minutes to ensure the hardboiled eggs are.

3. Remove the eggs and put them a few mins before peeling in an ice bath.

4. Scatter the eggs in 2 and suck the yolks out.

5. Put eggs white into a tray.

6. Add tabasco, homemade mayonnaise and herbal salt, then pound the yolks with a fork.

7. Apply the mixture to the egg whites, using two spoons, and finish with one shrimp or a slice of smoked salmon.

7. No-bread Keto Breakfast Sandwich

(Ready in about 15 mins |Serving 2| Difficulty: Easy)

Per serving: Kcal 354, Fat:30g, Net Carbs:2g Protein:20g

Ingredients

- Butter 2 tbsp

- Eggs 4

- Salt & pepper

- Smoked deli ham 1 oz

- Cheddar cheese 2 oz

Instructions

1. Add butter and set over medium heat to a frying pan. Add the eggs and fried them over. Season with salt & pepper.

2. For each "sandwich," use the fried egg. Put the ham/cold cuts/pastrami / next onto each plate, then the cheese is added. Round off with a fried egg on each plate. If you would like the cheese to melt, keep it in the tub on low heat.

3. If you like, add a few drops of Worcestershire sauce or Tabasco, and serve.

8. Low-Carb Baked Eggs

(Ready in about 15 mins |Serving 1| Difficulty: Easy)

Per serving: Kcal 498, Fat:35g, Net Carbs:2g Protein:41g

Ingredients

- Ground beef 3 oz

- Eggs 2

- Shredded cheese 2 oz

Instructions

1. To 200 ° C (400 ° F), preheat the oven.

2. Arrange a fried mixture of ground beef in a serving platter. Then build two holes and knock the eggs into them with a hammer.

3. Sprinkle over with shredded cheese.

4. Bake in the oven for around 10-15 mins, until the eggs are cooked.

5. Let them cool down for a bit.

Chapter 2. Snacks & Side Dishes Recipes

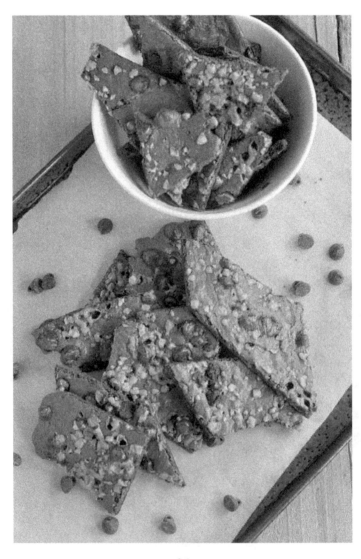

Snacks
9. Keto Brownie Bark

(Ready in about 45 mins | serving 12 | Difficulty: medium)

Per serving: kcal 98, Fat: 8.3g, net carbs: 4.3g, Protein: 2.4g

Ingredients

- Almond flour 1/2 cup

- Baking powder 1/2 tsp

- Salt 1/4 tsp

- Egg whites 2 large

- Swerve sweetener granular 1/2 cup

- Cocoa powder 3 tbsp

- Instant coffee (optional) 1 tsp

- Butter melted 1/4 cup

- Heavy whipping cream 1 tbsp

- Vanilla 1/2 tsp

- Chocolate chips sugar-free 1/3 cups

Instructions

1. Oven preheated to 325f, and line a baking sheet with bakery release paper. Greaseproof paper to the bakery release paper.

2. Stir together all the baking powder, almond powder as well as salt in the small bowl.

3. Beat a white egg in the large mixing bowl until they're frothy. Beat until smooth in cocoa powder, sweetener & instant coffee, after which beat in softened butter, vanilla & cream. Beat in a mixture of almond meal until it's combined.

4. Spread batter over nonstick baking paper in a 12 by 8-inch rectangle. Stir the chocolate morsels.

5. Bake and set for 18 mins, until puffed. Now remove it from the oven and turn off the Oven and allow to cool for 15 mins.

6. To cut it into 2inch squares, use a filet knife or pizza cutter but don't separate. Return it to a hot oven for 8-10 mins to gently crisp up.

7. Remove, allow it cool down & then split it into squares.

10. Homemade Nutella Sugar-Free

(Ready in about 20 mins | serving 6 | Difficulty: easy)

Per serving: kcal 158, fat: 18.23g, net carbs: 4.74g, Protein: 3.33g

Ingredients

- Hazelnuts toasted & husked 3/4 cup

- Melted coconut oil or avocado oil 2-3 tbsp

- Cocoa powder 2 tbsp

- Powdered Swerve sweetener 2 tbsp

- Vanilla extract 1/2 tsp

- Pinch salt

Instructions

1. Crush hazelnuts in a mixing bowl or a full power blender until deftly ground & start clumping together.

2. Add two spoonfuls of oil & continue to whip until the nuts become smooth in the butter. Add rest of the ingredients, then mix until well mashed. If the combination is quite thick, then add an extra table cubic oil.

11. Snickerdoodle Truffles

(Ready in about 20 mins | serving 12 | Difficulty: easy)

Per serving: kcal 150, Fat: 14g, net carbs: 13g, Protein: 3g

Ingredients

- Almond flour 2 cups

- Swerve, confectioners 1/2 cup

- Tartar cream 1 tsp

- Ground cinnamon 1 tsp

- Salt 1/4 tsp

- Butter melted 6 tbsp

- Vanilla extract 1 tsp

Instructions

Truffles

1. Mix almond powder, swerve, tartar cream, cinnamon & salt in the large bowl. Incorporate softened butter & vanilla extract until the dough gets together. If dough becomes too crumbly to scrape together, add a spoonful of water & stir it.

2. Scoop out dough through the circular tablespoon and press just a few times in your

palm to help hold it together. After this, shape it into a ball. Put on a baking tray lined with paraffin paper & repeat it with existing dough.

12. Low-Carb & Gluten-Free Coconut Chocolate Chip Cookies

(ready in about 30 mins | serving 20 cookies | Difficulty: easy)

Per serving: kcal 238, fat: 21.59g, net carbs: 8.18g, Protein: 4.39g

Ingredients

- Almond Flour 1 1/4 cups

- Unsweetened coconut finely shredded 3/4 cups

- Baking powder 1 tsp

- Salt 1/2 tsp

- Butter softened 1/2 cup

- Swerve sweetener 1/2 cup

- Yacon syrup 2 tsp

- Vanilla extract 1/2 tsp

- Large egg 1

- Chocolate chips sugar-free 1/3 cup

Instructions

1. Oven preheated to 325f, & line the large parchment or polyurethane liner cooking sheet.

2. Whisk the almond powder, cocoa powder, baking soda as well as salt with each other in a mixing bowl.

3. Softened butter with the molasses & erythritol in the large bowl. In vanilla & egg beat until just combined. Hit through flour mixture until it's mixed with dough. Mix in free of sugar chocolate morsels or hand - made chocolate-free chips

4. Shape the dough into the 1/2inch pieces and put it on a cookie sheet 2-inch apart, push every ball to 2 1/2inch thick with the heel of one's hand.

5. Bake twelve to fifteen mins, until just brown & hardly firm to touch.

6. Remove it from the oven and allow the pan to cool.

Side Dishes
13. Bread and dried Sun Tomato – Low-Carb

(Ready in about 1hour 30 mins |Serving 12| Difficulty: Easy)

Per serving: kcal 262, Fat:23g, Net Carbs:3g Protein:8g

Ingredients

- Salted melted butter 3/4 cup

- Eggs 4

- Almond milk unsweetened 1/2 cup

- Zucchini shredded 1/2 cup, crushed dry in a paper towel

- Dried sun tomatoes chopped 2 tbsp

- Almond flour 2 cups

- Coconut flour 1/4 cup

- Baking powder 4 tsp

- Granulated sugar 1 tsp

- Xanthan gum 1/2 tsp

- Kosher salt 1 1/4 tsp

- Dried oregano 1/2 tsp

- Dried parsley 1/2 tsp

- Garlic powder 1/4 tsp

- Ground asiago cheese 1/2 cup

Instructions

1. Oven Preheated to 350 ° C (F)

2. In a grinder, mix (wet ingredients) together with all the butter, peas, almond milk, zucchini & dried tomatoes, then blend for around thirty seconds or almost smooth.

3. Blend all the (dry ingredients) coconut flour, almond flour, baking soda, sweetener, xanthan gum, cinnamon, oregano, parsley, garlic powder in the med sized bowl and combine with a fork until well mixed without lumps.

4. place the dry ingredients into the wet ingredients and combine with a fork until it creates a smooth batter and absorbs the dry ingredients.

5. Mix in cheese made in Asiago.

6. In a greased loaf tin/twelve muffin cups, spoon your batter.

7. Bake for 1 hr. at 350 ° (F) while creating a loaf.

8. When creating muffins, bake at 350 ° (F) for twenty to twenty-five mins.

14. Keto Egg Fast Fettuccini Alfredo

(Ready in about 20 mins |Serving 1| Difficulty: Easy)

Per serving: kcal 491, Fat:47g, Net Carbs:2g Protein:19g

Ingredients

For the pasta:

- Eggs 2

- Cream cheese 1 oz

- Pinch salt

- Pinch of garlic powder

- Black pepper 1/8 tsp

For the sauce:

- Mascarpone cheese 1 oz

- Grated parmesan cheese 1 tbsp

- Butter 1 Tbsp

Instructions

For pasta:

1. In a grinder, add your eggs, cheese, cream, spice, garlic powder & pepper. Put into an 8 x 8 tray greased with butter. Bake eight minutes at 324 or before you just set. Remove& allow it to cool for five mins. Use a spatula to release the "pasta" sheet from the pan nicely. Turn it over and slice all into one/eight-inch thick pieces with a fine knife. Unroll softly, then put back.

For the sauce:

1. In a shallow cup, add the mascarpone, the parmesan cheese, and butter. 30 Second microwave on big. Click. Then click. Microwave another 30 seconds on big. Whisk until smooth again (this will take a minute since the sauce may be scattered-keep whisking, and it will come back together.) Add the pasta to the hot sauce and mix gently. Serve directly with freshly ground black pepper.

15. Grilled Eggplant Salad

(Ready in about 42 mins |Serving 6| Difficulty: Easy)

Per serving: Cal 183, Fat:10g, Net Carbs:23g Protein:4.3g

Ingredients:

- Thin Asian Eggplants 6

- Olive oil 1T to brush eggplants

- Fresh-& salty ground black pepper to season eggplants

- Grape tomatoes 1 cup

- Crumbled Feta 1/2 cup

Dressing ingredients:

- Fresh basil leaves 2/3 cup

- parsley leaves 1/3 cup

- large sliced garlic cloves 2

- Dijon mustard 1 t

- capers 3 t

- lemon juice 2 t

- additional-virgin olive oil 1/4 cup

Instructions

1. Heat up until med-high to BBQ.

2. Clean the eggplant if possible, then cut two ends. Cut the eggplant lengthwise, brown on both sides with olive oil, then top with salt & pepper upon its cut side

3. Put the cut side eggplant on your plate, then cook until you see some nice grill grates (about 5 to 7 mins).

4. Turn eggplant & cook for about five mins on the other hand, or until the eggplant is softened & very well browned.

5. Take the eggplant off from the cutting board & let It cool. Cut the tomatoes(grape) in half to make the beautiful dressing as the eggplant cool down.

6. Clean and turn as needed, dry out the basil & parsley leaves.

7. Choose the garlic cloves, then use a food processor with a steel blade to slice basil, peters, & ginger.

8. Apply the Dijon, capers, as well as lemon juice, then mix until the ingredients combine well; Now add the olive oil & stir it for thirty seconds.

9. Split it into pieces about one inch across, if the eggplant is treatable sufficiently.

10. Mix the eggplant & tomato halves nicely in a bowl and blend to coat the ingredients in a bread dressing (around 1/4 cup). For just another moment, save the remainder of dressing; too many things are perfect.

11. Apply a crumbled Feta & enjoy it.

16. Pan-Roasted Radishes (Low-Carb & Gluten-Free)

(Ready in about 60 mins | Serving 2| Difficulty: Easy)

Per serving: kcal 122, Fat:12g, Net Carbs:2.75g Protein:1g

Ingredients

- Quartered radishes 2 cups

- Butter 2 tbsp

- Lemon zest 1 tbsp

- Chopped chives 1 tbsp

- Pepper & salt to taste

Instructions

1. Melt the butter on a big, sauté pan. Apply the radishes, turn them down to protect. Cook over med heat for around ten mins, sometimes stirring until its color changes to golden brown & softened. Remove it from heat and add the lemon zest & the chives. Top it with salt & pepper.

2. Alternatively, you should roast these in olive oil at 374 degrees (F) oven for about 35 mins. And add seasonings that you'd like.

Chapter 3. Keto Poultry Recipes

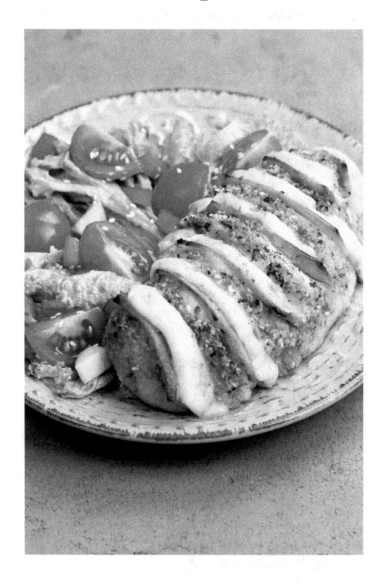

17. Low-Carb Keto Hasselback Chicken

(Ready in about 40 mins |Serving 4| Difficulty: Easy)

Per serving: Kcal 112, Fat:34g, Net Carbs:1g Protein:24g

Ingredients

- Boneless chicken breasts 4

- Hot capicola 3 ounces

- Fine provolone cheese 3 ounces

- Olive oil 2 tbsp

- Kosher salt 1 tsp

- Ground black pepper 1/4 tsp

- Garlic powder 1/2 tsp

For the pepperoncini cream sauce:

- Mascarpone cheese 4 ounces

- Butter 1 tbsp

- Kosher salt 1/4 tsp

- Minced pepperoncini 2 tbsp

- Chopped basil 2 tbsp

Instructions

1. Oven preheated to 375 °.

2. Trim some fat or gristle on chicken breasts, then create slices three/four of the direction through the upper edge of every breast, about one inch apart. The amount of slices differs according to the size of every chicken breast.

3. Place the olive oil over a sheet pan of med size & apply salt, pepper & garlic powder.

4. Push every chicken breast on both sides thru the olive oil & seasoning combination until completely coated, then put the pieces facing up onto the sheet pan.

5. Split the capicola pieces in two, then turn into thin strips the provolone cheese.

6. Put 1 piece of provolone strip in each of the chicken breasts pieces.

7. Bake for twenty-five mins or until the chicken is completely cooked.

8. Take the chicken from your oven & move it to plates/serving tray.

To the cream sauce pepperoncini:

1.   In   a   med sized   bowl, mix the (cheese) mascarpone   &   butter, then microwave it for thirty sec.

2. Stir together it strongly until smooth – that can take a few minutes.

3. Mix in the salt as well as the pepperoncini.

4. Serve hot on over chicken, and if desired, garnish with great basil & some more pepperoncini.

18. Spinach Stuffed Chicken Breasts

(Ready in about 25 mins | Serving 6| Difficulty: Easy)

Per serving: Kcal 434, Fat:16g, Net Carbs:3g Protein:6g

Ingredients

- Chicken breasts 3

- Spinach cooked chopped frozen 8 oz

- Feta crumbled 3 oz

- Cream cheese 4 oz

- Diced garlic 1 clove

- Salt 1/4 tsp

- Pepper 1/8 tsp

- Olive oil 1 tsp

Instructions

1. Oven preheated to 230 degrees Celsius.

2. In a med sized bowl, combine the sliced frozen spinach, feta, cream, garlic & half the salt.

3. Slice chicken breast into a pocket. If you're not sure well how to make a pocket into chicken

without cutting a pocket into the hand, try this: position the chicken flat on even a chopping board one at a time, then place a large spatula flat on the upper of the breast. Make sure you press down the spatula firmly enough to keep your chicken in place. To achieve this, you will need to drill its edge of the spatula into the meat just a bit. Add the two/three-knife through way into the side of the chicken's thickest part, & cut off the thinnest part, preventing before cutting through; you need a pocket, never a flap.

4. The spinach & cheese combination is separated into 3 parts & roll into thinner logs. Stuff every log into the chicken breast pocket you've made. Sprinkle with salt & pepper.

5. In an ovenproof pan placed over med-high heat, heat the olive oil, after which apply the stuffed chicken, side down "row." cook for five min, after this turn over the chicken.

6. Place the frying pan in the oven and cook for ten mins. If the chicken breasts are exceptionally thinner, cook for 2-5 mins more.

19. Keto Chicken Shawarma

(Ready in about 20 mins |Serving 4| Difficulty: Easy)

Per serving: Cal 274, Fat:16g, Net Carbs:0g Protein:35g

Ingredients

For the chicken shawarma:

- Boneless chicken breast 2 pounds

- Ground coriander 1 tsp

- Ground cumin 1 tsp

- Ground cardamom 1 tsp

- Ground turmeric tsp

- Ground cayenne pepper 1/2 tsp

- Smoked paprika 1 tbsp

- Garlic powder 1/2 tsp

- Onion Powder 1/2 tsp

- Kosher salt 1.5 tsp

- Ground black pepper 1/4 tsp

- Lemon juice 2 tbsp

- Olive oil 3 tbsp

For the tahini sauce:

- Tahini paste 2 tbsp

- Olive oil 2 tbsp

- Water 3 tbsp

- Lemon juice 1 tbsp

- Chopped garlic 1 clove

- Kosher salt 1/2 tsp

Instructions

For shawarma chicken:

1. Mix well all the ingredients for the marinade in a large mixing bowl.

2. Apply your chicken to marinade & flip to ensure it is thoroughly coated.

3. Marinate overnight for the most flavorful results-otherwise two hours would do it.

4. Grill preheated to 260 ° C.

5. Roast a chicken on the grill for around four mins each side over direct heat.

6. Take the chicken from the grill and allow to rest for ten mins.

7. Pick in and eat with your option of tahini sauce & side dishes.

For sauce tahini:

1. Mix all of the ingredients in a small bowl of tahini sauce.

2. Mix good until smooth.

20. Chicken with Bacon Mustard Sauce

(Ready in about 30 mins |Serving 3| Difficulty: Easy)

Per serving: Cal 677, Fat:37g, Net Carbs:7g Protein:73g

Ingredients

- Dijon mustard 1/3 cup

- Paprika 1/4 tsp

- Salt 1/4 tsp

- Black pepper 1/8 tsp

- Chopped strips bacon "8" uncooked

- Chopped onion 1 cup

- Olive oil 1 tbsp

- Boneless & skinless chicken breasts 2 1b

- Chicken broth 1 1/2 cups

Instructions

1. In a tiny bowl, mix Dijon mustard, paprika, salt & pepper to form a paste. Distribute the paste equitably over the chicken breasts on both sides. Put on aside.

2. Fry chopped bacon in a large pan on med-high heat until it changes to brown. Take away the plate, having left a pan with bacon fat. Add minced onion to the same pan, & fry in bacon fat until softened. Remove with bacon from the same plate.

3. Add one tbsp of olive oil to the same pan, now empty and hot. Roast chicken breast at med heat, on each side for around 1.5 mins. The chicken isn't going to be done as you continue to cook it in the next step. Remove your chicken onto a plate.

4. Add 1 & 1/2 cups of chicken broth to the same pan, bring to boil, and scrape the bottom of the saucepan. Apply bacon & onions in the back, then mix well. Add the chicken breast back, lower the heat & cook for around 15 to 20 mins, flipping the chicken, until the chicken breast is completely cooked & no pink now in the middle.

Chapter 4. Pork, Beef & Lamb Recipes

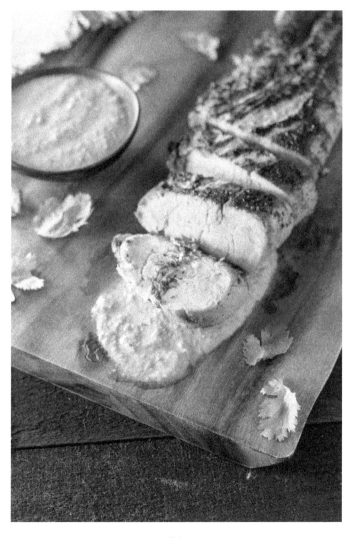

Pork

21. Keto Marinated Pork Tenderloin

(Ready in about 20 mins | Serving 4 | Difficulty: Easy)

Per serving: kcal: 258, Fat: 19g, Net Carbs: 1g, Protein: 24g

Ingredients

- Cut into 2 long pieces of pork tenderloin 1lb.
- Olive oil ¼ c
- Greek seasoning 2 tbsp
- Red wine vinegar 1 tbsp
- Lemon juice 1 tbsp
- Salt & pepper

Ingredients list for Greek Seasoning:

- Garlic powder 1 tsp
- Dried oregano 1tsp
- Dried basil 1tsp
- Dried rosemary ½ tsp
- Dried thyme ½ tsp
- Dried dill ½ tsp

- Cinnamon ½ tsp

- Parsley ½ tsp

- Marjoram ½ tsp

*Mix all the ingredients well enough & use an airtight container to place them.

Instructions

1. Mix the olive oil, vinegar, lemon juice & seasoning in a big zip lock container.

2. Put the 2 pieces of pork tenderloin in the container and marinate in the fridge overnight.

3. Place the pork over medium heat in a frying pan. Place the pork with one side and roast. Then by using tongs, turn the pork into a good browning on every side.

4. Continue to turn the pork until the inner temp reaches 145 F/63 C (control using a meat thermometer).

22. Keto Herbs Pork Tenderloin

(Ready in about 20 mins | Serving 2 | Difficulty: Easy)

Per serving: kcal: 627, Fat: 49g, Net Carbs: 4g, Protein: 44g

Ingredients

For the herb paste

- Pine nut 2 tbsp

- Chopped garlic cloves 3

- Fresh basil leaves 1 c

- Fresh parsley ½ c + 2 tbsp

- Nutritional yeast 2 tbsp

- Olive oil 5 tbsp

- Juice of 1 lemon

- salt >> *to taste*

For the pork

- Pork tenderloin 14 oz

- Salt & ground black pepper

- Olive oil 1 tbsp

- Reserved herbs paste 3 tbsp

Instructions

1. Begin by toasting pine nuts in a heavy, dry skillet to create the herb paste. Take out the crispy pine nuts and apply the garlic, basil, nutritional yeast flakes, fresh parsley, and olive oil to a mini food processor. Combine to make a perfect paste, scraping many times across the sides of the container. Season with salt & lemon juice to taste. Place on the side.

2. Preheat oven to 410 ° F (210 ° C) for pork.

3. Season the pork tenderloin on both sides with salt and freshly ground black pepper. In a non-stick pan heat the olive oil & brown the tenderloin at both sides. Remove from heat and let it cool down a little bit. Using a palette knife or thin silicone spatula until cool enough to treat, then spread the stored herb paste over the pork tenderloin on both sides. Put tenderloin with a well-equipped cover in a casserole dish & cook in the oven for 12-15 mins or until cooked to your taste.

4. Remove from oven and enable it to cool before sliced and served. Serve with some extra herbs paste if needed.

Beef

23. Garlic Herbs Butter with Filet Mignon

(Ready in about 15 mins | Serving 8 | Difficulty: Easy)

Per serving: kcal: 350, Fat: 29g, Net Carbs: 0.16g, Protein: 20g

Ingredients

- Butter 2tbsp

- Fresh rosemary ½ tbsp

- Fresh thyme ½ tbsp

- Minced garlic clove 1

- Filet mignon (8 oz)

- Sea salt>>to taste

- Black pepper>>to taste

Instructions

1. Put half of the butter together (1 tbsp, 14 g), rosemary, thyme, and garlic. (Sprinkle with a slight amount of sea salt while using unsalted butter.) Form into a log and cool before the last phase.

2. To 400 °F, preheat the oven.

3. Trim some connective tissue along beef tenderloin margins. The filets are liberally seasoned on both sides with salt & black pepper.

4. In medium-high pressure, pressure the cast iron skillet until the skillet is heavy. Melt the rest of the butter in the skillet (1 tablespoon, 14 g).

5. Add those fillets. Sear on either hand for two minutes, without turning them anymore.

6. Move the skillet to the oven, which is preheated. Bake for ideal doneness stage. For a 2 in (5 cm) thick filet, that is five minutes for uncommon, 6 minutes for medium unusual, 7 minutes for medium-well, or 8 mins for medium good. Using a meat thermometer to verify the correct temperature for medium well-125 °F (52 ° C) for normal, 130 °F (54 ° C) for medium fine, 140 ° F (60 ° C) for average, and 155 ° F (68 ° C). The temperature rises by an additional 5 degrees F when resting.

7. Take the filets from the oven and move to a tray. Cover each one of them with 1/2 tbsp (7 g) of herb butter (cut the butter log into four pieces and place one on each steak). Before cutting, let steaks rest for 5 mins.

24. Low-Carb - Hunan Beef

(Ready in about 12 mins | Serving 4 | Difficulty: Easy)

Per serving: kcal: 317, Fat: 21g, Net Carbs: 4g, Protein: 24g

Ingredients

- Coconut aminos 2 tbsp

- Sherry cooking wine 2 tbsp

- Arrowroot powder 1 tbsp

- Flank steak 1 lb.

- Avocado oil 3 tbsp

- Crushed Dried Thai chile peppers 2

- Minced garlic cloves 2

- Ground ginger ½ tsp

- Black pepper ¼ tsp

Instructions

1. Stir the coconut aminos, cooking water, and arrowroot powder together in a medium dish. Attach the sliced beef to brush and flip. Put back for 30 minutes to marinate.

2. Heat avocado oil to high heat in a broad wok. Stir the beef in and fry for almost a min.

3. Connect Thai chili peppers, sliced garlic, ground ginger & black pepper. Fry for another minute.

4. Serve with cooked broccoli (please cut out the Parmesan). Where appropriate, garnish with chives & sesame seeds.

Chapter 5. Fish & Seafood

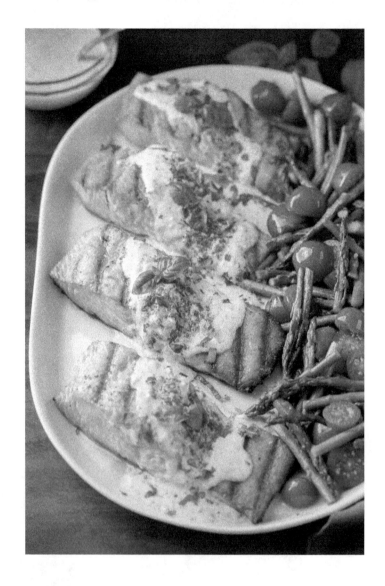

Fish

25. Baked Salmon with Pesto – Keto

(Ready in about 20 mins | Serving 4 | Difficulty: Easy)

Per serving: Kcal: 1025, Fat: 88g, Net Carbs: 3g, Protein: 52g

Ingredients

- Green sauce

- Green pesto 4 tbsp

- Mayonnaise 1 c

- Full-fat Greek yogurt ½ c

- Salt & pepper>> to taste

- Salmon

- Salmon 2 lbs.

- Green pesto 4 tbsp

- Salt & pepper>>to taste

Instructions

1. In a greased baking dish, put the salmon skin-side down. Sprinkle the pesto on top, and salt and pepper.

2. Bake in the oven for around 30 minutes at 400 ° F (200 ° C), or until the salmon flakes easily with a fork.

3. In the meantime, mix the sauce ingredients, pesto, mayonnaise & yogurt.

26. Keto Salmon with Pesto & Spinach

(Ready in about 25 mins | Serving 4 | Difficulty: Easy)

Per serving: Kcal: 893, Fat: 77g, Net Carbs: 3g, Protein: 45g

Ingredients

- Salmon 1&1/2 lb.

- Mayonnaise or sour cream 1 c

- Green pesto or red pesto 1 tbsp

- Grated parmesan cheese 2&1/2 oz

- Fresh spinach 1 lb.

- Butter or olive oil 1 oz

- Salt and pepper>> to taste

Instructions

1. To 200 ° C (400 ° F), preheat the oven.

2. Grease a baking dish with half the butter or oil. Salt & pepper the salmon fillets and put in the prepared baking tray, skin-side down.

3. Combine the mayonnaise, parmesan cheese, and pesto and spread over the salmon.

4. Bake for 15–20 mins, or until the salmon is fully completed & easily flakes with a fork.

5. Meanwhile, sauté the spinach in remaining butter or oil until wilted, around 2 minutes.

6. Serve with the oven-baked salmon right away.

27. Keto Salmon Pie

(Ready in about 55 mins | Serving 4 | Difficulty: Medium)

Per serving: Kcal: 1056, Fat: 97g, Net Carbs: 6g, Protein: 34g

Ingredients

- Pie crust

- Almond flour ¾ c

- Sesame seeds 4 tbsp

- Coconut flour 4 tbsp

- Ground psyllium husk powder 1 tbsp

- Baking powder 1 tsp

- Pinch of salt

- Olive oil or coconut oil 3 tbsp

- Egg 1

- Water 4 tbsp

Filling

- Smoked salmon 8 oz

- Mayonnaise 1 c

- Eggs 3

- Fresh dill, finely chopped 2 tbsp

- Onion powder ½ tsp

- Ground black pepper ¼ tsp

- Cream cheese 5 oz

- Shredded cheese 5 oz

Instructions

1. Preheat an oven to 175 ° C (350 ° F).

2. Put the pie dough ingredients in a food processor equipped with a plastic pastry blade. Pulse before the mixture forms a mass. If you don't have a food processor, use a fork to mix the dough.

3. Fit a sheet of parchment paper into a spring-shaped 10-inch (23-cm) pan. (This allows it a cinch to cut until it is cooked.)

4. Grease the fingertips or a spatula and press the dough softly into the spring-shaped plate. Pre-bake the crust for 10–15 minutes or until light brown.

5. Combine all the filling items, excluding salmon, and pour in a pie crust. Add salmon & bake for 35 minutes or until golden brown.

6. Cool for a couple of minutes, then serves with salad or other veggies.

Seafood Recipes
28. Creole Butter Grilled Lobster's Tails– Keto

(Ready in about 18 mins | Serving 4 | Difficulty: Easy)

Per serving: Cal: 213, Fat: 13g, Net Carbs: 2g, Protein: 23g

Ingredients

- Raw lobster tail 4

- Salted butter ½ c

- Fresh garlic minced 2 tsp

- Creole seasoning 1 tbsp

- Fresh parsley Chopped 2 tbsp

Instructions

1. In a small bowl, add the garlic, softened butter, parsley, and Creole seasoning and with a fork, mix well until blended. Put aside for keeping soft at room temp.

2. Prepare the grilling lobster tails and cut in two or cut through the bottom and removing the meat from the shell.

3. Preheat the grill to around 400 ° F, put downside the meat of the lobsters for around 3 mins over direct heat.

4. Turn over the tails, then with the soft Creole butter, gently baste the meat.

5. Cook for another 3 or 4 mins, or until the meat is cooked completely.

6. Serve with extra Creole butter melted instantly, if desired.

7. Keep in the refrigerator excess butter for about one week or about three months in the freezer.

29. Low-Carb Lobster Chowder

(Ready in about 35 mins | Serving 6 | Difficulty: Medium)

Per serving: Cal: 210, Fat: 15g, Net Carbs: 4g, Protein: 14g

Ingredients

- Chopped raw bacon 4

- Chopped onion ½ c

- Salted butter ¼ c

- Lobster broth 2 c

- Cauliflower florets raw 2 c

- Almond milk unsweetened 3 c

- Cooked chunks of lobster 2 cups

- Kosher salt tsp 1.5

- Black pepper ¼ teaspoon

- Garlic powder ¼ teaspoon

- Xanthan gum ¼ tsp

- Cider apple vinegar 2 tbsp

- Cointreau 3 tbsp

- Parsley chopped 2 tbsp

- Butter 1 tbsp

Direction

Lobster broth:

1. Combine shells & body from a lobster to a medium saucepan, and four water cups. Bring to boil, reduce heat, simmer for 15 minutes. Strain out the liquid. For this dish, you would need broth 2 cups. The remainder may be discarded or freeze.

Chowder:

1. Cook the butter, bacon, and onion over less heat in a wide saucepan for 3 to 4 mins until onions are soft & cooked through the bacon is not crispy.

2. Add cauliflower and lobster broth. Cover and cook for 5 to 8 mins, just until cauliflower is soft but does not fall apart.

3. Almond milk is added & gently heat for 2 to 3 mins. Don't ever boil.

4. The lobster is added & gently heat for further 3 minutes.

5. Remove broth 1/2 cup and whisk xanthan gum to a tiny bowl. Add the chowder back and stir before fully combined.

6. Stir the cider apple vinegar, parsley, Cointreau, & 1 tablespoon butter. Keep stirring until the butter is thoroughly melted and incorporated.

7. Seasoning to taste & adjust to the preference.

Chapter 6. Meatless Meals

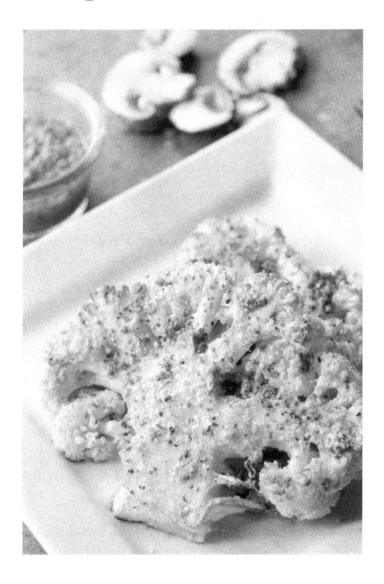

30. Parmesan Cauliflower Steak

(Ready in about 30 mins | Serving 4 | Difficulty: Easy)

Per serving: Cal: 386, Fat: 13.5g, Carbs: 56.8g, Protein: 15.3g

Ingredients

- Large head cauliflower 1

- Butter 4 tbsp

- Urban accents manchego and roasted garlic seasoning blend 2 tbsp

- Parmesan cheese ¼ c

- Salt and pepper to taste

Instructions

1. Preheat oven to 400 ° C

2. Remove cauliflower leaves

3. Slice the cauliflower into 1-inch steaks lengthwise around the core.

4. Melt butter in a microwave and blend along with seasoning mixture to make a paste

5. Brush mixture over the steak and season with pepper and salt to taste

6. Heat a non-stick pan over medium heat and position steaks with cauliflower for 2-3 minutes until nicely browned

7. Flip over gently and repeat

8. Put chopped steaks on a lined baking sheet

9. Bake steaks with cauliflower in the oven for 15-20 mins until golden & tender

10. Sprinkle with cheese & serve.

31. Creamy Low-Carb Cilantro Lime Coleslaw

(Ready in about 10 mins | Serving 5 | Difficulty: Easy)

Per serving: Kcal: 53, Carbs: 3.2g

Ingredients

- Coleslaw bagged 14 oz

- Avocados 1.5

- Cilantro leaves ¼ c

- limes, juiced 2

- garlic clove 1

- Water ¼ c

- Salt ½ tsp

- Cilantro>> to garnish

Instructions

1. Place the garlic and cilantro in a food processor and cook until sliced.

2. add in the lime juice, avocado, and water. Pulse Up to nice and creamy.

3. Take the avocado mixture out and combine it with the coleslaw in a large bowl. It'll be a bit thick, but it'll be nicely covering the slaw.

4. For better performance, refrigerate to soften the cabbage for a few hours before eating.

32. Low-Carb Cauliflower Hummus

(Ready in about 30 mins | Serving 6 | Difficulty: Easy)

Per serving: Cal: 141, Fat: 14g, Net Carbs: 3.5g, Protein: 2g

Ingredients

- Raw cauliflower florets 3 c

- Water 2 tbsp

- Avocado or olive oil 2 tbsp

- Salt ½ tsp

- Whole garlic cloves 3

- Tahini paste 1.5 tbsp

- Lemon juice 3 tbsp

- Raw garlic cloves crushed 2

- Olive oil 3 tbsp

- Kosher salt ¾ tsp

- Smoked paprika & olive oil for serving

Instructions

1. Combine the cauliflower, water, 2 tbsp of avocado or olive oil, 1/2 tsp of kosher salt, and 3 entire cloves of garlic to a safe microwave dish. Microwave for approximately 15 minutes-or before softened or when color is intensified and darkened.

2. Put the mixture of cauliflower into a magic bullet, mixer, or food processor and combine. Add the tahini paste, lemon juice, 2 raw cloves of garlic, 3 tbsp of olive oil, and 3/4 tsp of kosher salt. Usually, blend until smooth. Seasoning to taste and adjust when required.

3. Place the hummus in a bowl and drizzle with extra virgin olive oil & a sprinkle of paprika to serve. Using thinly sliced tart apples, sticks of celery, fresh radish chips, or other vegetables to dip.

33. Roasted Caprese Tomato with Basil's Dressing

(Ready in about 35 mins | Serving 4 | Difficulty: Easy)

Per serving: Kcal: 198, Fat: 15g, Carbs: 9g, Protein: 8g

Ingredients

- Ripe tomatoes 6

- Olive oil 1 tbsp

- Balsamic vinegar 2 tbsp

- Salt & pepper>> to taste

- Thin slices mozzarella 6

- Basil leaves 6

For the dressing

- Garlic clove 1

- Small handful fresh basil

- Juice of a half lemon

- Olive oil 2 tbsp

- Salt & pepper>> to taste

Instructions

1. To 180 ° C/350 ° F preheat the oven.

2. Slice the tomatoes into half and put them on a non-stick baking sheet, cut side up.

3. Drizzle over olive oil & balsamic & season with salt & pepper, then top with mozzarella & basil leaves, the 4 bottom halves. Add the tomatoes tops.

4. Roast until the skins are blistered & the tomatoes are tender, for 20-25 minutes.

5. Blitz all the ingredients in a tiny food processor to produce the sauce before the basil is finely chopped.

6. Serve the drizzled tomatoes with crusty bread dressing.

Chapter 7. Soups, Stew & Salads

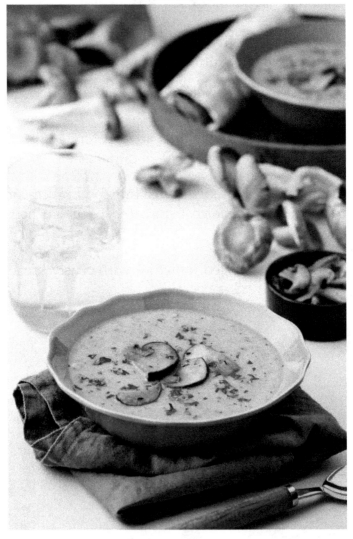

Soups

34. Wild Mushroom Soup

(Ready in about 30 mins | Serving 4 | Difficulty: Easy)

Per serving: Kcal: 468, Fat: 45g, Net Carbs: 11g, Protein: 6g

Ingredients

- Butter 4 oz

- Shallot 1

- Portobello mushrooms 5 oz

- Oyster mushrooms 5 oz

- Shiitake mushrooms 5 oz

- Garlic clove 1

- Dried thyme ½ tsp

- Water 3 c

- Chicken or vegetable bouillon cube 1

- Heavy whipping cream 1 c

- Celery root ½ lb.

- White wine vinegar 1 tbsp

- Fresh parsley

Instructions

1. Clean, trim & chop mushrooms & celery root. Peel and chop the garlic and onion thinly.

2. In a heavy-bottomed saucepan, sauté the chopped vegetables in butter over medium heat until golden brown. Save a few tablespoons of mushrooms.

3. Add thyme, vinegar, bouillon cube & water & bring to a boil. Reduce heat and allow to cook for fifteen min or until soft.

4. Add the cream and mash with an immersion blender until the desired consistency is reached. Serve with finely chopped parsley & a few pieces of mushroom on top.

35. Philly Cheesesteak Soup – Low-Carb

(Ready in about 40 mins | Serving 6 | Difficulty: Medium)

Per serving: Kcal: 356, Fat: 24g, Net Carbs: 4g, Protein: 29g

Ingredients

- Butter 3 tbsp

- Sliced red onion 1/2

- Green bell pepper, sliced 1

- Mushrooms, sliced 4 oz

- Salt and pepper>> to taste

- Deli roast beef, chopped 1 lb.

- Beef broth 4 c

- Cream cheese softened 4 oz

- Shredded white cheddar cheese 6 oz

- Provolone cheese 3 oz

Instructions

1. Melt the butter in a large saucepan over medium heat. Add the onions and sauté until tender but not browned for about 5 minutes. Stir in the chili peppers & mushrooms and sprinkle with salt & pepper. Cook for another 3 to 4 minutes, until tender.

2. Add the beef to the frying pan and mix well. Stir in the broth & cook for 10 minutes.

3. Place the cream cheese in a blender & add about 1/4 of the hot broth from the saucepan. Mix until smooth and the cream cheese has melted. Pour the mixture back into the saucepan and stir until melted.

4. Preheat the broiler. Place the soup in safe bowls or ramekins over the oven & top with a piece of provolone. Set on a baking sheet & place under the broiler until the cheese is melted & bubbly, 2 to 4 mins.

5. Serve immediately.

Stew

36. Italian Beef Stew with Zucchini, Mushroom & Basil- Paleo

(Ready in about 1 hr. 40 mins | Serving 8 | Difficulty: Medium)

Per serving: kcal: 348, Fat: 14g, Carbs: 10g, Protein: 47g

Ingredients

- Chuck roast cut into cubes 2 lb.

- Olive oil 5 tsp

- Salt & ground black pepper >> to taste

- 2 can beef broth 14 oz

- 2 cans petite diced tomatoes with juice 14.5 oz

- Italian herb blend 1 t

- Ground fennel seed 1 tsp

- Medium onion, chopped 1

- Large green pepper chopped 1

- Small zucchini, ends trimmed and then cut into half lengthwise

- Mushrooms cut in thick slices ½ lb.

- Chopped fresh basil 4 t

- Balsamic vinegar

Instructions

1. Trim the roast with chuck & cut into cubes. In a large non-stick pan, heat the 2 teaspoons of olive oil and brown the beef cubes over medium to high heat until the meat is browned on all sides, about 10-15 mins.

2. Add salt & fresh-ground black pepper to the meat as it cooks. Don't rush this step; browning adds flavor to the meat.

3. Stir the browned meat into the stew pot.

4. Add 1 can of beef broth to the frying pan & cook for a minute, scraping with a turner to loosen the brown bits of meat that stick to the pan, then add that can of beef broth to the stew pot together with the other.

5. Stir & add the diced tomatoes with juice, Italian Herb Blend, and ground fennel.

6. Turn to medium-low heat and simmer for 60 minutes, or slightly longer, if the meat doesn't feel tender once you pierce it with a fork.

7. While the stew simmers, peel & chop the onion, and cut off the green pepper, and chop stem & seeds. Cut the ends off the zucchini, lengthwise cut in half & thick slices.

8. Wash mushrooms or rinse in a sink colander & blot dry, & cut mushrooms in thick slices or 1/2 slices,

9. When the stew is ready to finish, heat 1 tsp. Olive oil In a frying pan, add onions & green peppers and cook over med-high heat for a few minutes, then add to the stew.

10. Heat the second tsp of olive oil, add the zucchini, & cook until both sides are slightly browned, then add to the stew. Then add the slices of the mushrooms, cook until their liquid is released and start browning, then add to the stew.

11. Simmer for about fifteen minutes, then add the chopped basil & cook for a few more minutes.

12. Serve hot, with a good quality balsamic vinegar to sprinkle on at the table if you wish.

Salads

37. Keto Broccoli Slaw – Low-Carb & Gluten-Free

(Ready in about 35 mins | Serving 6 | Difficulty: Easy)

Per serving: kcal: 110, Fat: 10g, Net Carbs: 2g, Protein: 2g

Ingredients

- Olive oil 1 tbsp

- Sugar-free mayonnaise 1/3 c

- Apple cider vinegar 1&1/2 tbsp

- Dijon mustard 1 tbsp

- Granulated sugar substitute 2 tbsp

- Celery seeds 1 tsp

- Kosher salt ½ tsp

- Black pepper ¼ tsp

- Bagged broccoli slaw 4 c

Instructions

1. Whisk together the olive oil, mayonnaise, apple cider vinegar, mustard, sugar substitute, celery seeds, salt, & pepper in a large bowl until

completely combined. Add the slaw on broccoli. Toss to coat. Serve chilled.

38. Salad Green Bean

(Ready in about 27 mins | Serving 6 | Difficulty: Easy)

Per serving: Cal: 232, Fat: 20g, Carbs: 13g, Protein: 5g

Ingredients:

- Green beans fresh 1 lb.

- Sliced palm hearts 2 cups

- Kalamata olives/black olives 3/4 cup, sliced in half and drained

- Bell pepper red diced roasted 1 cup

- Feta cheese crumbled 1/2 cup

- Black pepper fresh ground

Dressing ingredients:

- Balsamic vinegar 1 T

- lemon juice fresh-squeezed 2 T

- Olive oil 1/3 cup

- Lemon zest 1 tsp.

- Fresh oregano chopped 2 T

- Fresh basil chopped 2 T

Instructions

1. Trim green beans end.

2. Cut the beans into about 2″ long pieces.

3. Steam beans in a big pot having a lid tight-fitting or a vegetable steamer (electric), using a steamer insert until they are some tender-crisp.

4. When beans are tender as you would like them, take off the steamer and immediately plunge into an ice water bowl to halt the cooking.

5. Remove the beans to a colander and allow them to drain and cool for about 15 mins, then spread the beans on towels on paper and then blot dry.

6. While the beans cook, slice and drain the palm hearts, drain & red peppers chop, drain and cut olives in half, then measure the feta.

7. Combine lemon juice, balsamic vinegar, olive oil, chopped oregano, lemon zest & chopped basil & process until the herbs are chopped very thinly, and the dressing is well mixed.

8. Combine drained beans and sliced palm heart, olive halves, & red pepper chopped to assemble the salad.

9. To moisten salad, add dressing as required and gently combine.

10. Add the feta cheese & stir to make the feta barely mix.

11. Grind black pepper & serve straight away.

12. This can keep inside the refrigerator for several days but bring the leftovers to room temp before serving.

39. Anti-Pasta Cauliflower Salad – Low-Carb & Gluten-Free

(Ready in about 75 mins | Serving 8 | Difficulty: Easy)

Per serving: Cal: 102, Fat: 8g, Carbs: 4g, Protein: 3g

Ingredients

- Chopped Raw cauliflower 2 c

- Chopped Radicchio ½ c

- Chopped Artichoke hearts ½ c

- Chopped fresh basil 1/3 c

- Grated parmesan ½ c

- Chopped Sundried tomatoes 3 tbsp

- Chopped Kalamata olives 3 tbsp

- Minced Clove Garlic1

- Balsamic vinegar 3 tbsp

- Olive oil 3 tbsp

- Salt & pepper

Instructions

1. First, cook five minutes in the microwave the chopped cauliflower. Do not add any seasoning or liquid to it. Simply spread and zap it on the safe microwave platter. Let cool down the cauliflower while the further ingredients are prepared.

2. In a medium bowl, combine the artichoke heart, radicchio, basil, parmesan, olives, sundried tomatoes, & garlic.

3. Whisk the vinegar and olive oil together in a smaller bowl, then pour over salad. Toss it to coat, and sprinkle with salt & pepper. Can be chilled or served at room temperature.

Chapter 8. Brunch & Dinner Recipes

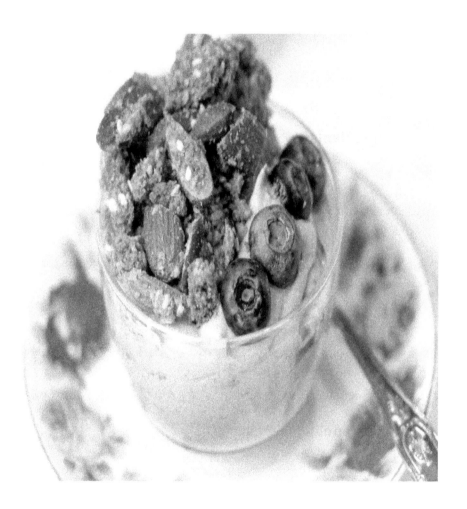

Brunch
40. Low-Carb Ginger and Licorice Granola

(Ready in about 25 mins | Serving 6 | Difficulty: Easy)

Per serving: Kcal 413, Fat: 33g Net Carbs: 9g, Protein: 18g

Ingredients:

- White 1 egg

- Chopped almonds 4½ oz.

- Sesame seeds 1 oz.

- Coconut oil 2 oz.

- Coconut 2½ oz.

- Almond flour ¾ cup

- Licorice powder 2 tsp

- Ground ginger 2 tsp

- Pinch salt

Instructions

1. To 150 ° C (300 ° F), preheat the oven.

2. Beat the white egg until smooth.

3. Mix in diced almonds and dry products.

4. Using the fingertips to work in the butter until the texture is even and the dough is one clump.

5. Break the granola in pieces onto the baking dish. 15–20 mins to put in the oven.

6. Turn around cautiously after three mins. Without fire, the Nuts can become crispy. It is going to take some 15–20 min.

7. Place in a securely packed jar at the refrigerator.

8. Serve with Greek yogurt full fat or a strong cream.

41. Keto Eggs Benedict

(Ready in about 25 mins | Serving 4 | Difficulty: Easy)

Per serving: Kcal 577, Fat: 46.4g, Net Carbs: 6g, Protein: 29g

Ingredients (English muffin)

- Coconut flour 1/4 cup

- Eggs, beaten 4

- Canned coconut milk 1/4 cup

- Baking soda 1/2 tsp

- Salt 1/2 tsp

Ingredients (hollandaise sauce)

- Egg yolks 3

- Water 1 1/2 tbsp

- Cold grass-fed butter (pieces small) 1/2 cup + 2 tbsp

- Salt

- Lemon juice 2 tsp

Ingredients (poached egg)

- Smoked salmon wild-caught 6 ounces

- Pastured eggs 8

- Lemon juice or apple cider vinegar 1 tbsp

- For garnish thinly sliced chives

Instructions:

1. First, cook the muffins in English. Whisk all muffin ingredients together in a small cup until smooth.

2. Divide the batter equally into four medium ramekins that are suitable for fire. Bake for 5-10 minutes at 350 degrees, or until an inserted toothpick comes out clean.

3. Prepare the Dutch sauce. Pick up one pinch of water with a small pan. Hold water over medium-high heat to a boil, then decrease to a low simmer.

4. In a medium glass cup, incorporate egg yolks and water that will stay on top of the saucepan without dropping in or hitting the bath. Place the bowl over the pan and whisk the egg mixture vigorously until it lightens and thickens (approximately 1-2 minutes).

5. Gradually combine the butter in bits, enabling them to melt one by one.

6. Remove risotto from heat and whisk until it is fully smooth, putting it back on the cooling casserole if required to hold it soft. Season

with lemon juice and spices. Pour sauce into a thermos to maintain warmth until hot.

7. Using poached eggs. Carry a water-filled saucepan to simmer. Reduce the flame to a soft simmer.

8. Crack one egg in a pinch container.

9. Stir water in a loop in the clockwise direction using a spoon to create a whirlpool in the pot core.

10. When whirlpool has developed, scatter the egg carefully into the middle of the whirlpool so that egg whites wrap around the yolk as they turn. Cook 5 minutes. (If you are comfortable with poaching eggs and have a fairly big grill, you will cook up to four at once.)

11. Remove eggs from the pot using a slotted spoon and put them on a paper towel to clean. Repeat as required, before poaching of all eggs.

12. Play Benedict keto chickens. Break the English muffins and toast thinly and add two bits of muffin to each pan. Cover each slice with a slice of smoked salmon, a poached egg, a hollandaise sauce, and a chives sprinkling. Serve forthwith.

42. No-Fail Instant Pot Soft-Boiled Eggs

(Ready in about 2 mins | Serving 2 | Difficulty: Easy)

Per serving: Kcal 71, Fat: 46.4g, Net Carbs: 0g, Protein: 6g

Ingredients

- Eggs 2

- Water 0.33cup

Instructions

1. Place the metal trivet inside your Instant Pot

2. Place eggs over the trivet. Up to 1 dozen eggs can be cooked

3. Load 1 cup of water to the saucepan.

4. Put the cover onto the Instant Pot, testing the sealing of the tube.

5. Click Button and change the duration of high pressure to 2 minutes.

6. Prepare a bowl of ice water as the eggs cook.

7. As soon as the Instant Pot beeps, relieve pressure right away.

8. Remove the cover and put each egg in the ice water tub, using tongs.

9. Peel the eggs gently, break, and serve after 2 or 3 minutes.

Dinner
43. Keto Pork Aphelia

(Ready in about 6 hours 15 mins | Serving 4 | Difficulty: Medium)

Per serving: Kcal 758, Fat: 59g, Net Carbs: 7g, Protein: 40g

Ingredients

- Red onions 2

- 1 whole garlic

- Red wine ¾ cup

- Olive oil ½ cup

- Coriander seed 2 tbsp

- Dried thyme 2 tsp

- Black pepper 2 tsp

- Ground cinnamon 2 tsp

- Pork shoulder 3 lbs.

- Salt 1 tbsp

Instructions

1. Peel the red onions and carve them into small wedges. Break the cloves of garlic in two. Add all of the marinade components

together. Place a wide freezer bag in a smaller freezer bag & apply half the mixture of onions to the container.

2. Rinse the collar of pork, rinse it well, and sauté it with garlic. Place the collar inside the freezer bag & pour over the marinade. Push all of the air out of the jar, close off the bag, and put it in a tub. Keep the bowl in the fridge for at least 12 hours, ideally more than this.

3. Preheat up the oven to 125 ° C (260 ° F).

4. Layer the beef, the remaining onion mix & marinade in a casserole dish that is suitable for the oven. Cover it with a tight-fitting lid & position the dish about 5 or 6 hours in the lower part of the oven. The meat is cooked in an electronic slow cooker on the picture; this turned out to be incredibly juicy and tasty. If you use a slow cooker, meat would be ready in around 8-12 hours if set to medium, although it all depends on the slow cooker model that you are using.

5. Pull the beef apart with two forks to cut, then completely blend with the gravy. Taste salt and change. Serve with low-carb toast, garlic butter, and coleslaw on this recipe.

44. Bacon-Wrapped Keto Meatloaf

(Ready in about 85 mins | Serving 4 | Difficulty: Medium)

Per serving: Kcal 1032, Fat: 90g, Net Carbs: 6g, Protein: 47g

Ingredients

Meatloaf

- Butter 2 tbsp

- 1 onion

- Ground beef 1½ lbs.

- Whipping cream ½ cup

- Shredded cheese 2 oz.

- 1 egg

- Oregano 1 tbsp

- Salt 1 tsp

- Black pepper ½ tsp

- Sliced bacon 7 oz.

Gravy

- 1¼ cups whipping cream

- ½ tbsp soy sauce

Instructions

Meatloaf

1. To 200 ° C (400 ° F), preheat the oven.

2. Melt butter in a pan over medium heat. Add onion & fry until crispy, but not crisped, then set leave to cool.

3. In a tub, add ground beef. Connect all the other products and the fried onion, except bacon. Mix well, just stop overworking it, or the final product may be too thick.

4. Form into a loaf & put in an oiled baking platter. Place the bacon loaf in.

5. Bake for 45 mins in mid-oven. If the bacon starts overcooking until the pork is cooked, cover it with aluminum and reduce the heat a little bit. If the bacon doesn't seem entirely cooked, roast the meatloaf for another 5 minutes.

Gravy & serving

1. Keep the juices in the baking tray that have gathered and use to produce the gravy. In a smaller frying pan, add the liquids with the milk.

2. Bring to a boil & lower the heat and enable it to simmer for 10 to 15 minutes before the correct

consistency is reached. Using a little soy sauce to try if you like.

3. Serve with honey, salt, and pepper or some side dish of your choice of freshly cooked broccoli.

Chapter 9. Desserts & Drinks Recipes

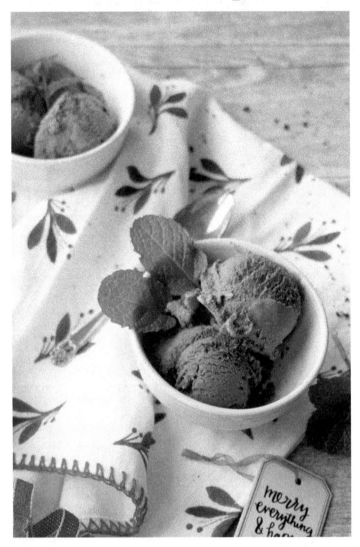

Desserts

45. Low-Carb Peppermint Mocha Ice Cream

(Ready in about 30 mins | Serving 6 | Difficulty: Easy)

Per serving: Kcal 390, Fat: 38g, Net Carbs: 4g, Protein: 6g

Ingredients

- Heavy whipping cream 2 cups

- Sugar-free dark chocolate 2 oz.

- Egg yolks 6

- Powdered erythritol ⅔ cup

- Instant coffee powder 2 tbsp

- Vanilla extract 2 tsp

- Salt ½ tsp

- Food grade peppermint extract 1 pinch

- Liquid sweetener 6 pinches

Instructions

1. In a heavy saucepan over low heat, heat the heavy cream, stirring with a whisk.

2. Add the chocolate and continue stirring until the chocolate has melted. Add the egg yolks. Continue whisking on low heat until just warmed.

3. Add the powdered sweetener and the instant coffee powder and whisk until completely dissolved. Continue heating, constantly whisking, until the custard thickens, about 10 minutes.

4. When the custard coats the back of a wooden spoon or reaches 140°F (60°C) on a candy thermometer, remove the pan from the heat. Do not allow the mixture to warm to over 140°F, or the eggs will begin to cook.

5. Stir in the vanilla extract, salt, and peppermint. Taste and add the liquid sweetener. Place in the refrigerator to cool.

6. When cool, churn the ice cream mixture in an ice cream maker following the manufacturer's directions until it reaches your desired consistency.

46. Keto Chocolate Cake with Chocolate Glaze

(Ready in about 40 mins | Serving 8 | Difficulty: Easy)

Per serving: Kcal 321, Fat: 30g, Net Carbs: 22.4g, Protein: 6.5g

Ingredients:

- Coconut flour 1/2 cup

- 5 eggs

- Coconut oil 1/2 cup

- Coconut cream 1/2 cup

- 2 tsp vanilla extract

- 4 tbsp sweetener

- 1/2 cup cocoa powder

- Salt pinch

- Coconut oil for smearing

- Chocolate glaze ingredients:

- Coconut cream 1 cup

- 1 tbsp ghee

- 1 tsp vanilla extract

- 1 tbsp cacao powder

- 1 tbsp erythritol

- Salt pinch

Instructions:

1. Preheat the oven around 350 ° C. Grease butter, ghee to an 8-inch round cake tray.

2. Whisk the egg whites until a frothy consistency emerges.

3. Mix the remaining ingredients for the chocolate cake in a small dish. Then insert egg white gently into the mixture.

4. Place flour into a tray for coffee. Bake for 25 minutes, or until clean comes out a knife inserted into the cake middle.

5. Prepare glaze as the chocolate cake starts to cool. Put all glaze components in a low-heat saucepan and whisk vigorously to mix.

6. Place chocolate glaze over the cake into a glass container and drizzle. Serve the chocolate cake hot, or keep it covered in the fridge or freezer.

47. Low-Carb Keto Cupcakes Recipe

(Ready in about 32 mins | Serving 2 | Difficulty: Easy)

Per serving: Kcal 66, Fat: 5g, Net Carbs: 7g, Protein: 1g

Ingredients

- Coconut flour 1/3 cup

- Cocoa powder 1/2 cup

- Powdered erythritol 1/4 cup

- 1 tsp baking powder

- 1/2 tsp baking soda

- 1/4 tsp salt

- 4 eggs

- 1 tsp vanilla extract

- Stevia extract 8 drops

- 4 tbsp olive oil

- Almond milk 1/2 cup

Instructions

1. Preheat the oven around 350 F. Prepare a muffin tray with cupcake liners by greasing.

2. Whisk the coconut flour, chocolate powder, baking powder, erythritol, baking soda, and salt together in a medium dish.

3. Create a well in dry mixture core. Add olive oil, vanilla essence, stevia & almond milk. Mix when the components are blended properly. Let sit for 5-8 minutes.

4. If the paste becomes smoother in consistency, then you would like to feel free to apply 2 Teaspoons of water to the batter before the ideal consistency is met.

5. Spoon 2 Batter spoons inside each container. Bake for 20 minutes and clean before toothpick falls out.

6. Frost with low-calorie frosting and enjoy.

Drinks

48. Turmeric Ginger Lime Tea Recipe

(Ready in about 5 mins | serving 1 | difficulty: easy)

Per serving: kcal 13, Fat: 0g, carbs: 1.8g, Protein: 0g

Ingredients

- 1 lime which is sliced into large slices

- 1 small turmeric root that is peeled and sliced into small pieces

- 1 piece of ginger the same size as the turmeric root that is peeled and sliced into small pieces

Instructions

1. Put 1 lime slice in a big teapot, along with all pieces of turmeric & ginger.

2. Load teapot with hot water and heat.

3. Let the tea take 5 minutes to brew.

4. Enjoy steam & then chill the iced variant of the tea.

49. Cacao Coffee Recipe

(Ready in about 30 mins | serving 1 | difficulty: easy)

Per serving: kcal 335, Fat: 19g, Net carbs: 10g, Protein: 8g

Ingredients

- Cacao nibs 1 cup

- Boiling water

- Gelatin ½ tsp

- Just a splash of coconut oil ted

- Just a pinch of cinnamon powder

Instructions

1. Preheat the oven to 350 ° c.

2. Place cacao nibs on the baking sheet, in a thin film.

3. Put in oven and enable to cook 15 to 18 min.

4. Remove from the frying pan and allow cool. Place in a packed box.

5. You'll need 1 tbsp of cacao nibs for 1 cup of hot water to create a cup of coffee.

6. Place coffee grinder with the cacao nibs and trigger 4 times for 2 sec each. Holding down the button will bring you a substance. Take the boiling water and put it in the French press.

7. Let them seep for five to eight minutes.

8. Put your gelatin & cold-water splash in your cup, then stir with a spoon.

9. Pour the coffee into your cacao and apply the coconut oil & cinnamon. You should save the ground and dry it out for 8 minutes in the oven at 300, then grind it into fine flour & use it in baking.

50. Keto & Low-Carb Pumpkin Spice Latte

(Ready in about 3 mins | serving 1 | Difficulty: easy)

Per serving: kcal 183, Fat: 17g, Net carbs: 4g, Protein: 2g

Ingredients

- 3/4 cup unsweetened almond milk

- 1/4 cup cold brew

- 1 tbsp California gold nutrition, MCT oil

- 1/4 tsp pumpkin pie spice

- 1/2 tsp vanilla extract

- 3 tbsp swerve, the ultimate sugar replacement, granular

- 2 tbsp pumpkin puree

Instructions

1. Apply all ingredients to the mixer and add for 30 - 60 seconds.

2. Cover with additional pumpkin pie seasoning, and whipped cream.

Conclusion

Losing weight quickly is one of the goals of most people who suffer from overweight, obesity, or pathologies such as diabetes, hypertension, or hypercholesterolemia, among others. The problem is that, in the middle of the eagerness to see those extra kilos diluted, some people fall into restrictive diets that eliminate entire groups of macronutrients.

One of these fashionable diets that, among other things, turns out to be effective in the short term, is the ketogenic or Keto diet. Many health professionals, especially endocrinologists, nutritionists, or bioenergeticians, implement ketogenic diets in weight loss centers.

What Are the Advantages of the Keto Diet?

In short, you have the following:

- **Metabolic Flexibility:** The ability to change metabolism in an agile way.
- **Autophagy:** The ketone bodies you produce when you are on keto activate autophagy.
- **Satiety and Hunger Control:** The lack of sugars and ketone bodies makes you (sometimes literally) forget to eat.

- **Improves Your Cholesterol:** In general, your lipid profile improves.
- **And a Couple of Other Less Obvious Benefits:**
    o If you follow a keto diet, you will inevitably learn to know and value what each type of food brings you, and you will take control over this facet of your life.
    o If you were one of those people who organized your life around food, the keto diet will drastically change your relationship with food (for the better).